Invisalign

Questions
and
Answers

Everything You Need to Know

by

Dr. Janet Stoess-Allen

Park Avenue Orthodontics, LLC

935 Park Avenue. Suite 102,
New York, NY 10028
(212) 452 – 2777

www.ParkAveOrtho.com
info@parkaveortho.com

Dr. Stoess-Allen

About Dr. Janet Stoess-Allen

Dr. Janet Stoess-Allen graduated with honors from the University of Kentucky, with a Bachelor of Science degree in Dental Hygiene. After a five-year practice as a dental hygienist, she enrolled in the University of Louisville's School of Dentistry to complete an advanced dental education. Thereafter, she enrolled in New York University's College of Dentistry, where she completed a two-year orthodontic residency.

Dr. Stoess-Allen is a member of the American Association of Orthodontists (AAO), the Northeast Society of Orthodontists (NESD), the American Dental Association (ADA), the New York Dental Society, and the Women's Academy of Dentistry (WAD). She volunteers her time and expertise by providing orthodontic assessments and management consultation to charitable organizations such as the Little Baby Face Foundation, which offers treatment worldwide to children who have facial and dental deformities. She also participates actively in the Make a Wish Foundation and in the Smiles Change Lives organization.   Who's   Who   recently   named   her Orthodontist of the Year.

Dr. Stoess-Allen and her husband live in Manhattan. They are the proud parents of their son, Zach.

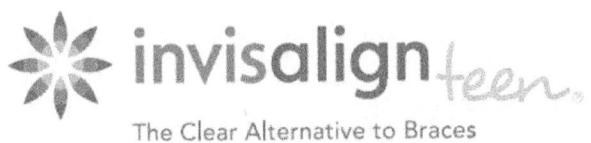

The Clear Alternative to Braces

Answers to Frequently Asked Questions

How visible is Teen Invisalign?

Invisalign aligners are made of a virtually invisible plastic. In fact, your child will be surprised to find out how many people won't even notice they are going through orthodontic treatment.

Do you find that teenagers are responsible enough to wear Teen Invisalign?

Invisalign Teen Aligners feature compliance indicators which fade over time with wear so that the doctor can monitor patient cooperation. In my practice teenage Invisalign patients are usually our most responsible and compliant patients and they love the fact that people cannot tell that they are wearing anything in their mouths at all during treatment.

What if my child loses or misplaces his aligners occasionally?

Invisalign offers up to 6 free replacement trays free of charge if misplaced or lost. This is something that is not offered to adults. However, in my practice, we have found that our teen patients are very responsible and rarely lose an aligner.

My child has a lot of crowding. Will Teen Invisalign work for all situations?

Invisalign Teen has been proven to be effective across a very broad range of cases, from mild problems to severe. Your orthodontist will be able to tell you immediately if your child is a candidate.

When using Teen Invisalign, will my child need more frequent appointments than if she were wearing braces?

Invisalign Teen can result in fewer appointments by virtually eliminating potential emergency visits that are more common with treatment using traditional braces.

I know that there are many dietary restrictions when wearing braces. Is the same true when using Teen Invisalign?

Invisalign Teen allows your teen to eat all of their favorite foods whenever wanted because the aligners are removable. Braces are not removable so the diet is much more restricted.

With braces it is difficult to keep the teeth completely clean. Is the same true with Teen Invisalign?

Teens using Invisalign can easily keep brushing and flossing their teeth as usual. The aligners are completely removable allowing them to brush and floss their teeth as prescribed by their orthodontist and dentist.

How does the price compare for Teen Invisalign and traditional braces?

In our practice, our prices for traditional orthodontic treatment using braces and using Teen Invisalign are very comparable. The same flexible payment plans are available for both methods of treatment.

I understand there may be a lot of emergency visits when using braces due to sharp wires or broken brackets. How does this compare to using Teen Invisalign?

With Teen Invisalign there is no worry about sharp brackets or wires cutting your teen's mouth as there are no brackets or wires. Invisalign Teen is made of a clear plastic material that is soft and also removable.

My child wore braces and it interfered with the musical instrument he played. Will the same be true with Teen Invisalign?

Whether your teen plays sports or a musical instrument, braces can often be cumbersome and interfere with instruments or sports mouthguards. There is no interference when using Teen Invisalign since it is removable. When playing instruments or playing sports, the Invisalign aligners can simply be removed so that they will not ever interfere with things teens enjoy doing. Invisalign Teen will help your teen focus on doing what they do best while being a teenager.

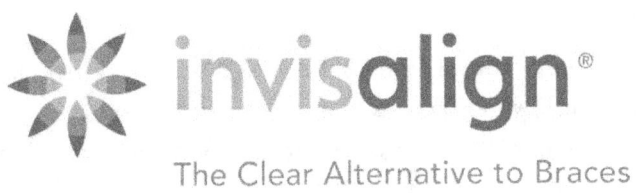

The Clear Alternative to Braces

Answers to Frequently Asked Questions

What are the advantages of Invisalign, and is there any disadvantage?

For a patient, the only disadvantage to treatment with Invisalign is the need to commit to wearing something in your mouth full time. But Invisalign's aligners are very thin, so they're unobtrusive after the patient has worn them for even just a day or two. As for the results, as long as the treating orthodontist writes the prescription specifically for Invisalign's laboratory technicians, Invisalign works beautifully, and the results are excellent. Compared to the price of traditional orthodontics, Invisalign is also very competitive and fair.

Does Invisalign work if you switch from regular braces?

Yes. Treatment for some patients will start with Invisalign and finish with braces, and in other cases, the reverse will be true. But in most cases, treatment with Invisalign alone is all that is required.

What is the difference in cost between Invisalign and braces?

The difference in cost between braces and Invisalign depends on the difficulty of the patient's particular situation. In my practice, orthodontic treatment and treatment time are usually very similar for Invisalign and for braces, and the price of treatment is similar too.

Is the price range about the same for Invisalign and Invisalign Teen?

For the regular Invisalign product, there are different product types, such as Invisalign Express 5, Invisalign Express 10, Invisalign Assist, and Comprehensive Invisalign, and they have different prices. For Invisalign Teen, there is just one product. In my orthodontic practice, the pricing for Comprehensive Invisalign and Invisalign Teen is very similar. In general pricing depends very much on the length of the required treatment, the difficulty of the particular case, and the type of product required for achieving the best overall result.

What is Invisalign Express, and how does it work?

Invisalign offers two Invisalign Express options, Invisalign Express 5 and Express 10. The numbers indicate the number of trays allowed for accomplishing the necessary or desired movement of your teeth. Invisalign Express 10 is for minor tooth movements, and Invisalign Express 5 is for very minor tooth movements. Both are for people who need only a few trays to reach their goals for tooth movement. For example, if you need only to close a small space between teeth or if you have only minimal crowding of your front teeth, you may be a candidate for an express product. Consult your orthodontist, who can evaluate your dental needs and recommend an Invisalign product to give you an optimal result.

I saw the Invisalign video on television, and Invisalign seemed to work like traditional metal braces. Will you please explain the difference between Invisalign and braces?

Because you wear Invisalign with attachments on particular teeth, the forces exerted by the clear plastic trays are very similar to the forces exerted by braces, so you can accomplish the same movements of teeth by using Invisalign instead of braces.

Will Invisalign cause a patient's bite to be off?

Whether a patient wears Invisalign or traditional braces, the bite will feel "off" temporarily. This is just to be expected. Patients often have a misconception that the bite should feel the same before, during, and after treatment. But when your teeth move during any sort of orthodontic treatment, they do not all move at the same time or at the same rate, so your bite may feel different during the actual tooth movement than it did before you started treatment. Eventually, the teeth catch up, and the bite should feel uniform and comfortable.

Does it take longer to correct an overbite with Invisalign?

It should not take longer to correct an overbite with Invisalign than with traditional braces. I have found in my orthodontic practice that an overbite often decreases more rapidly with aligners than with traditional braces.

Can Invisalign really correct an underbite?

Depending on an underbite's severity and on the jaw structure, it is quite possible to correct the underbite using Invisalign. One must understand that for boys, growth of the mandible may continue until well into the twenties, and for girls, until a few years earlier. In some cases of underbite, one must consider the patient's age and level of growth when attempting to correct a "skeletal" discrepancy. Your orthodontist should be able to guide you in this determination.

Can Invisalign help correct a bad bite that is causing jaw asymmetry?

Yes. Invisalign is useful for nearly all orthodontic alignment issues. Often, with movement of the teeth into a normal arch formation, with proper leveling, aligning, and symmetry from side to side, the jaw will shift automatically to a more normal position. However, if an actual bony disfigurement is causing the jaw asymmetry, surgery may be necessary. Therein lies the difference between a dental problem on one hand and a skeletal problem or combined problem on the other hand.

Would Invisalign or Lumineers be better to correct widely spaced teeth and improve bite?

It is always better to align teeth properly using orthodontics rather than to mask an orthodontic problem using Lumineers, crowns, laminates, and so forth. Orthodontic treatment places teeth in a proper alignment, not only side by side, but also between upper and lower teeth. Only after completing the orthodontic tooth movement and correcting the occlusion should one do any cosmetic dental work such as crowns, laminates, or Lumineers. To maintain your teeth for life, it is best to correct your occlusion or dental relationships before doing any desired cosmetic work. For information on pricing, it is wise to consult both an orthodontist and a cosmetic dentist.

I am on my second to last trays of Invisalign and my bite feels very uncomfortable. When I asked my treating dentist about it, he said it was normal. My jaw hurts when I close my teeth together. What should I do?

When any healthcare professional treats you, it is important that you feel able to communicate your concerns and that you feel you are heard. The purpose of any orthodontic tooth movement is not only to achieve nice aesthetics, but more importantly, to provide an accurate, comfortable, and functional bite. If you feel that an orthodontic treatment is moving your teeth into an uncomfortable position, it is imperative that you voice your concerns to your orthodontist, and it is equally important that your orthodontist attempt to address them. Sometimes during orthodontic tooth movement, your bite will feel worse before it gets better, so it may be that you have to go through an uncomfortable time to get to a better bite. However, if the discomfort persists, and you are nearing the end of your treatment, you may need to have an alternate treatment plan devised by the orthodontist. Feeling that your lower jaw is being pushed back too far, for example, is a valid concern that needs to be discussed and addressed.

Is it normal for my bite to feel misaligned while I am wearing Invisalign?

When you begin using your first Invisalign trays, you may feel your bite changing, and the feeling may be awkward and uncomfortable. It is quite normal for your bite sometimes to feel out of alignment as you experience orthodontic tooth movement. As your teeth move, your bite may feel as if it does not fit together properly, and it may feel worse than it did before you began wearing the trays. This is quite normal. Depending on the alignment of your bite before you began treatment and the difficulty of the movement necessary to make your corrections, you may feel that your bite is "off" for some time. Patients with easier corrections will feel less discomfort with their bite than those who need drastic changes. Discuss your case with your orthodontist so that you have a complete understanding of what to expect as your teeth move. Upon completion of your treatment, your bite should feel very comfortable, as your teeth fall together into a normal occlusion. Be patient. Give your treatment time to progress, but be sure to discuss your discomfort with your orthodontist so that you can feel assured that it is normal for your case.

Do rubber bands and Invisalign work together, to correct the bite?

Wearing rubber bands (elastics) with Invisalign trays helps to correct a malocclusion (improper bite) in the same way that wearing them with braces does. The elastics slowly move the bite into a more acceptable position. It is very important to wear the elastics for the prescribed number of hours each day and to change to a fresh pair as often as prescribed. Light, continuous forces acting on the teeth and jaw are critical for achieving the best bite. When worn as the orthodontist directs, elastics are very effective.

Will my teeth shift considerably if I leave my Invisalign aligners out for a week?

If you are in an active state of tooth movement with Invisalign, the answer is YES, your teeth will shift if you don't wear your aligners for a week. Invisalign aligners are supposed to be worn for twenty hours daily for the optimal results. Light, continuous forces are most effective when moving teeth, so the interruption in treatment will disturb the natural progression and allow negative changes. If you commit to using Invisalign for your orthodontic tooth movement, be sure you are also committed to wearing the aligners as prescribed.

After completing the full treatment with Invisalign, how long do you need to use retainers?

One can never consider orthodontic tooth movement to be altogether stable. The teeth undergo changes just as the rest of the body undergoes changes from birth. The teeth will move if not retained, and the bottom front teeth are prone to the most noticeable movement. Retention should begin immediately after orthodontic treatment. After the completion of tooth movement using Invisalign, if a patient's retainers are removable, I recommend that the patient wear them full time for one to three months, and then wear them every night while sleeping (for about eight hours daily), doing so indefinitely.

What kind of retainer works with Invisalign?

Invisalign can make one set of retainers for you or a series of retainers called Vivera. Vivera retainers are very similar to the Invisalign trays although made of a somewhat stronger material. If you purchase Vivera, you will receive four retainers per dental arch.

I broke my retainer, after having it for twelve years. Could my teeth start moving again?

Changes occur to the body over the years as we age, and the teeth are no exception. Whether you have had orthodontic treatment or you have not, your teeth can move if not retained. Most people notice changes to their lower front teeth in the form of "crowding." I recommend to my patients that they wear retainers indefinitely after orthodontic treatment. Immediately after orthodontic treatment, I advise them to wear retainers every night while sleeping, for about two years. After the two-year period of nightly wear, I suggest that they continue to wear their retainers at least a few nights each week. I explain to them that they will be able to tell how often to wear the retainers based on how they feel when they are worn. For instance, if the retainers feel tight, and the teeth feel sore after the patient misses a few nights of wearing the retainers, the patient should wear them more frequently, since the teeth are trying to shift. However, if the patient wears the retainers, and they feel "passive," with no discomfort to the teeth, this may indicate that the patient can wear them less often. I do not ever tell my patients to stop wearing retainers, as there is always the possibility of the teeth shifting out of the desired position.

Why do I feel that my teeth are no longer touching, after wearing my retainer? My retainers do not cover my back molars.

The fact that your teeth are no longer touching, except for your back molars, indicates that you are wearing a retainer that does not cover all of your teeth. If the retainer is too short and does not cover your back molars, they can extrude, which will cause your bite to be open on all the teeth anterior to them. Maybe the retainer has broken or worn very thin on the back molars. Another reason the bite could open after orthodontic treatment is a tongue-thrusting habit. It is very important to visit your orthodontist to discuss the problem and to have your orthodontist diagnose it and remedy it. The sooner you visit your orthodontist to discuss your situation, the better.

I lost my Invisalign tray on day 7. Can I go on to the next one?

Depending on the severity of your orthodontic situation and your consistency in wearing your Invisalign aligners, it is possible that you could move on to the next set of aligners after you have worn them for 7 days. However, it is best to consult your orthodontist before making any decision to go on to the next set. If you are not ready, the orthodontist may be able to order new trays to replace the ones you lost.

Can I go on to my next Invisalign tray after less than two weeks, if my teeth fit in it?

Even though it may feel as if you can move on to a new tray after less than the full two weeks, I do not suggest that you do so. When tooth movement occurs too rapidly, there can be adverse effects such as bone loss or root resorption. It is best to follow the Invisalign guidelines.

On Tray 14 of my Invisalign treatment, I noticed that my right canine and both lateral incisors are no longer moving into place. Should I wear this aligner for longer than 2 weeks?

Whenever you have a concern that a tooth is not "tracking" properly or fully into an Invisalign tray and the desired movement is not occurring, consult your orthodontist. The orthodontist can show you a virtual model of your teeth (ClinCheck) that will show exactly what tooth movements should occur with each tray. Sometimes, teeth will move out of proper alignment before being brought into an ideal alignment. The approved ClinCheck will allow you to visualize all expected movements.

Do you have to wear upper and lower refinement trays?

One of the advantages when using Invisalign is that they offer something called refinements after all of the initial sets of trays have been worn. The reason for this is to "tweak" the final product. If there are any teeth that have not moved fully into the designated positions, your orthodontist can request up to three refinements at no extra fee. That is, of course, if you have been treated with the comprehensive Invisalign product. Be sure to ask your orthodontist about the different options that Invisalign offers before beginning your treatment. If you need or desire a refinement, then your orthodontist can make new impressions or a scan of your teeth and send it to Invisalign with requested changes. Shortly thereafter, Invisalign will send new trays to you to address any concerns and finalize your treatment. Your orthodontist should discuss the desired changes with you, so that all of your concerns are addressed. Many times, it is imperative to treat both upper and lower teeth in order to accomplish the requested changes. For instance, if a lower front tooth is slightly rotated, it may be necessary to change the position of an upper front tooth slightly in order to move the lower one properly. Therefore, it will be necessary for you to wear both upper and lower trays that are active. In such a scenario, if there is no need to move the upper tooth, and the lower tooth can be moved into the proper position on its own, Invisalign may send trays that actively move the lower teeth and trays that are passive (holding trays) for the upper teeth. Every situation is unique, and one must address it properly, so that you receive the best possible outcome.

Do I need to use Invisalign for both top and bottom teeth even if only the bottom teeth are crowded?

Invisalign does offer the option of treating just one dental arch treatment. However, I have found that it is not advisable. When you are changing the positions of teeth on one arch only, there will be a very large chance that, at the end of treatment, the treated arch will no longer occlude (fit) well against the opposing arch of teeth. I always advise my patients to consider dual arch treatment only.

I originally had sixteen aligners for the top teeth and fifteen for the bottom. Then I had more impressions taken for my top teeth and received nine more aligners. My front teeth have not moved in the way shown to me, and now my dentist has said there is nothing else he can really do. What can I do?

It sounds as if your dentist treated you as a full, comprehensive Invisalign case based on the number of trays you have received. It also sounds as if you have done a refinement after your initial sets of trays. One of the beauties of treatment as a full case with Invisalign is that Invisalign allows up to three refinements after the initial sets of trays are completed. You may want to ask your orthodontist about using additional refinements that you may be entitled to, if you desire more orthodontic change.

I've struggled with the first three aligners, sometimes wearing them only at night, but now I've been wearing them for twenty-plus hours per day for ten days, and it feels fine. Can I carry on with treatment if I stick to the twenty-two-plus hours, fourteen days per aligner?

Because you are in the early stages of treatment with Invisalign, if the aligners are seating fully (tracking), it should be perfectly fine to continue with treatment at your current twenty-two-plus hours per day for ten-to-fourteen days.

I have to have one of my front teeth removed, and they will be replacing it with Invisalign and a fake front tooth. My question is, will I be able to eat while wearing the top aligners?

You should always remove your Invisalign aligners when eating. If you are self-conscious because of a missing tooth, you might want to discuss the possibility of using a removable appliance with a false tooth attached, one that you can place in your mouth while eating. You may also be a candidate for temporary use of a Marilyn bridge, a bonded false tooth, during the Invisalign treatment. You should discuss all possibilities with your orthodontist before undergoing Invisalign impressions or scans.

I've had impressions taken for Invisalign, but now I need a filling. Will a filling affect the aligners' fit?

Any time a tooth is altered, it will affect the fit of the aligners. This may affect the overall outcome of your treatment with Invisalign. For the best possible results, it is very important that the Invisalign aligners fit snugly on all of the teeth. Therefore, I strongly suggest that you complete all necessary dental work before having impressions taken for Invisalign. Any dental work that can wait until after the treatment is completed should wait, so that the fillings, crowns, laminates, etc., can be completed on a good, stable occlusion. If you need to have a filling made before receiving your first Invisalign trays, you must inform your orthodontist, so that new impressions or scans can be taken and new trays made to fit your new dental work.

Does Invisalign have an age limit? I am 52 years old, and I would like to have orthodontic work done with Invisalign. Is it possible?

Invisalign has no age limit. As long as your periodontal (gum and bone) health is good, you should be able to use Invisalign. In my orthodontic practice, we have been able to use Invisalign with children as young as ten years old, and the eldest patient was in her eighties. Your orthodontist will tell you whether you are a good candidate.

I have finished Invisalign treatment that involved slight extrusion of my upper lateral incisors. Is it possible that my laterals will move back into my gums (re-intrude) now that I'm using only a retainer?

It is always possible for a tooth that has been extruded to intrude slightly after orthodontic tooth movement is complete. If you are concerned, you may want to discuss the use of a lingual bonded retainer for added stability.

How can I prevent Invisalign attachments from popping off when I grind my teeth at night? Can I use a bite guard on top of Invisalign?

Invisalign attachments do become dislodged sometimes. If it happens, I advise meeting with your orthodontist to have the attachment replaced. An attachment can break off from the tooth due to grinding or due to merely inserting or removing the aligners. If you are a "grinder," I do not recommend wearing a bite guard with the aligners.

What is the best way to clean my Invisalign trays? Do you recommend using an ultrasonic cleaner like those used with dentures?

I recommend cleaning Invisalign trays with a toothbrush and toothpaste in cool water. An ultrasonic cleaner used with the "crystals" recommended by Invisalign will also work very well.

Will Invisalign treatment work for someone with periodontal disease?

Depending on the severity of the bone loss and the angulation of the teeth's roots, Invisalign can be an excellent option even for someone who has had periodontal disease in the past. If you have been diagnosed with periodontal disease, you should be under the care of a periodontist, who specializes in treating the gum tissue and the supporting bone. After the periodontist has confirmed that the disease has been eliminated or is properly under control, you may be a candidate for orthodontic tooth movement using Invisalign.

What are Invisalign "buttons" and where are they attached?

"Buttons" or attachments are tooth-colored or clear filling material bonded to the front of certain teeth to aid the prescribed tooth movement. They are very important for the most accurate tooth movements, and patients become accustomed to them rather easily.

I wear Invisalign, and one of my buttons has broken off. I usually wear an elastic from that button, and I'm wondering whether I should take off the other elastic?

If you were advised to wear elastics on both sides, the forces should be symmetrical; so until the button is replaced, do not wear any elastics.

Can Invisalign close a gap between my teeth?

Invisalign works very well for you. You will need to undergo a thorough examination and have a treatment plan devised, with the spacing both between and behind your teeth taken into consideration. When treatment involves space closure, retraction of teeth is often required, and proper space must exist between the teeth and the opposing teeth in order to achieve the desired result.

Will extraction of wisdom teeth affect treatment with Invisalign?

In most cases, extraction of wisdom teeth should not affect treatment with Invisalign. If you are already in treatment using Invisalign, and you have your wisdom teeth extracted, you may need to have your aligners altered. Discuss all of the options with your orthodontist.

Can Invisalign Cause Ear Pain?

It is possible to experience ear pain when wearing Invisalign, but not probable. If you are on the first set of trays, and you feel ear pain during the early morning hours, you may be clenching your teeth when you sleep, and you may feel ear pain due to the clenching. I would suggest continuing to wear the trays, to learn whether the pain was just a one-time occurrence. After wearing the trays for a longer time, you may find that there are no negative side effects at all. If they do persist, visit your orthodontist to discuss the problems, which may be easily resolved.

Should I have bonding or use Invisalign for small teeth with spaces?

If your teeth are unusually small, merely closing the spaces may not be aesthetically appealing to you. However, if the spaces are narrow, and all of your teeth are smaller than normal, it may be perfectly acceptable for you to have the spaces closed. If some of your teeth are small, such as the front ones, while others are normal in size, you may want to have your teeth moved orthodontically to prepare for bonding or for placement of porcelain laminates, after the tooth movement is complete. You should discuss all of the options with your orthodontist.

Can a bite be repaired where teeth have been excessively filed?

It is possible to use Invisalign to extrude teeth or to intrude them. With the technological advances and new attachments that are available for use with Invisalign, we can produce many different tooth movements that were not possible in years past. It is true that Invisalign can apply a force to bring a shortened upper tooth down into better contact with its opposing tooth. One key item is the way your orthodontist writes the prescription to Invisalign for your particular case, and another is the proper placement of attachments and other aids used to achieve the extrusion of a tooth.

Will Invisalign work after jaw surgery?

You may be treatable with Invisalign even if you need jaw surgery. Many of the most sophisticated orthodontists who use Invisalign are using it even with patients who need orthognathic surgery. Be sure to discuss with your orthodontist whether you are a candidate for Invisalign even though you need some surgical correction.

Will Invisalign change face structure?

Whether treatment with Invisalign will change the structure and look of your face will depend on many factors. For example, if someone has very protrusive top teeth, often referred to as buck teeth, your profile may change for the better when you use Invisalign to retract those teeth. As another example, sometimes an orthodontist must expand both the upper and lower dental arches to align the teeth better and to relieve crowding. The expansion often produces a pleasant change in the lower face by giving the lips better support. The change in structure to which you refer is almost always a pleasant change and not a detraction. Most adults feel they have achieved results that are anti-aging after treatment using Invisalign.

Will Invisalign push up a wearer's upper lip?

The difference in thickness between Invisalign trays and braces is significant. Braces are thicker and bulkier, sitting a few millimeters out from the teeth. Invisalign trays are much thinner, and they sit very close to the surface of the teeth, covering the teeth like a glove. Invisalign trays will not push the upper lip out, as braces will. When you are wearing Invisalign, most people will never even know that you are wearing anything on your teeth.

What are Invisalign chewies?

Invisalign chewies are Styrofoam-like cylindrical pieces that help to seat your Invisalign aligners when you chew on them. It's like chewing a piece of gum. When you have finished using chewies, you can rinse them and reuse them.

If an Invisalign wearer does not use chewies every day, will it greatly delay alignment?

The most important time to use the chewies with Invisalign is when starting on a new set of trays. The purpose of the chewies is to seat the aligners fully, to allow optimal movement of your teeth. As long as the trays seat themselves properly, it is not important to use the chewies every day, but when you change to a new set of trays, the chewies will help to seat the aligners on your teeth as well as possible, to aid in achieving the best possible tooth movement.

Should I use Invisalign or just have veneers placed on my teeth?

When considering cosmetic dentistry, such as placing veneers on teeth, it is very important to assess the occlusion. Things to consider are the crowding of the teeth to be veneered, their mal-positions, the periodontal health of the teeth involved, the depth of the bite, and other factors. It is always best to place veneers or crowns on teeth that are in their best positions. For example, if veneers are to be placed on the bottom front teeth, it is very important that the overbite is not too deep, that the lower teeth are not too crowded, and that the health of the teeth to be restored is excellent. If there is crowding of the bottom teeth, it is always best to straighten the teeth orthodontically before having the cosmetic work performed. That way, you have the best chance of achieving an excellent, long lasting, and dentally healthy result.

Is Invisalign appropriate for teeth with permanent bridges and veneers?

It is very possible to move teeth that have veneers or bridges on them. While moving teeth connected by a bridge is certainly more difficult than moving individual teeth, it is possible, and it is done every day. You should consult an experienced Invisalign orthodontist who can explain to you the possibilities and limitations of tooth movement using Invisalign.

Can a veneer be straightened after it was installed out of line?

A tooth with a veneer attached can be moved and straightened using Invisalign. Since a veneer is just a cover on an existing tooth, it will move along with the actual tooth, no more and no less. But if the veneer was made to mask the poor position of the tooth, you may need to have a new veneer made after the teeth are properly aligned.

My dentist told me that my orthodontist made a retainer for me that does not work for me and it has caused my teeth to be misaligned. He also said that I wasted my money that I paid my orthodontist. Should I begin Invisalign treatment with this dentist?

The main purpose of using Invisalign or any appliances for orthodontic correction is to correct misaligned teeth. You mentioned that your dentist suggested that you wasted the money you paid to the orthodontist who made your "retainer." My first issue is that your dentist has planted an inappropriate thought in your mind by speaking unprofessionally about another dental colleague. Maybe the "retainer" that you speak of is actually a removable appliance that will make corrections to that overlapped tooth that you mention. I feel it is inappropriate for one dental professional to speak disparagingly to you, the patient, about the work of another dental professional. If your dentist does not know what your orthodontist's goal is for you or does not understand what treatment is being provided, it would be most professional for the dentist to contact your orthodontist (with your approval) to discuss your case. I would be wary of the motives of your dentist in this circumstance and would seek another opinion.

Are there any reasons that someone should not be treated with Invisalign?

Almost all orthodontic malocclusions are treatable using Invisalign. Due to the great advances in the Invisalign technology, orthodontists are now able to achieve amazing results using Invisalign. Historically, there were orthodontic problems that were difficult to correct using Invisalign alone, without using braces at all; however, due to the great technological advances, we are now using Invisalign to treat almost every orthodontic concern. Today, you should feel confident that you are a candidate for Invisalign and schedule a consultation with an orthodontist.

Why should I have my Invisalign treatment done by an orthodontist versus a general dentist?

Treatment with Invisalign, or any other orthodontic procedure, will involve tooth movement and repositioning through bone and soft tissue. To become an orthodontist one must complete dental school and then specialize for two to three years in the field of orthodontics. During those intense years of training to become an orthodontist, time is spent understanding the physiology of tooth movement, all associated effects on the roots of teeth, the surrounding bone, the relationship of the lower jaw to the skull, and the muscles of the head and neck. All of this is not learned in dental school.

When planning to have your teeth positioned differently, whether it is for cosmetics of for better function, it is always advisable to consult with and be treated by an orthodontist who is a specialist in tooth movement. When using Invisalign the orthodontist will be very proactive in writing a detailed prescription outlining exactly how your teeth should be moved, what attachments should be used for your particular tooth movement needs, and exactly what the result should be on the finish of treatment. The result of your treatment is dependent on your commitment to wear the Invisalign trays for the proper number of hours daily and also on the prescription that is written by your orthodontist to achieve ideal goals.

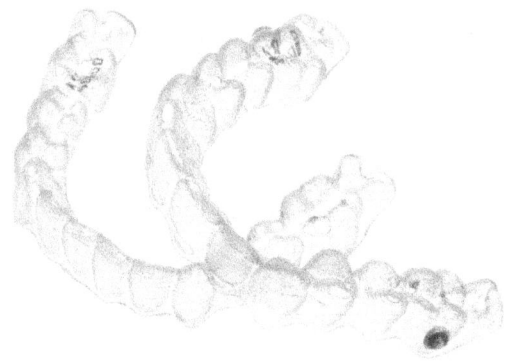